FAT VEGAN

Connie Rogers is a Certified Integrative Nutritional Health Coach

DISCLAIMER

The content of this book is for general instruction only.

Each person's physical, emotional, and spiritual condition

is unique. The instruction in this book is not intended to

replace or interrupt the reader's relationship with a

physician or other professional. Please consult your doctor

for matters pertaining to your specific health and dietary needs

Table of Contents

PREFACE

My Veganism began thirty years ago. I was neither a hippie or an activist, just sick, anemic and on several medications that didn't cure the problem. The diagnosis was ulcerative colitis and I spent many days in the hospital or at my doctor's office. Kidney stones was a side effect of taking Sulfasalazine and addiction was a side effect from Percocet, an opioid. After experiencing these side effects and the ulcerative colitis was not getting any better, I made the decision to use food as my medicine. My poisons were meat, caffeine and wheat. When I noticed I was still experiencing digestive issues, I cut out cheese. I listened to my body and never looked back. In fact, it prompted me to look for and make more creative fun plant-based recipes. I must have bought over a dozen new cookbooks at the time and felt creative in my own healing.

Seventeen years ago, one of my clients decided to become vegan. Her story began with addictions to cigarettes, caffeine, (soda and coffee) french fries, ice cream, hamburgers and a married boyfriend. Her desire to change her life happened when her boyfriend died in her arms from a heart attack. She swore there was something in that fast food crap that kept them both coming back for more, and she was right.

When you make that decision to become vegan for either health reasons (like mine) or to take a stand for cruelty to animals, or just to get the "crap" out, you begin an awareness about your food choices.

Ask yourself-What's your reason?

Are you concerned with breast or colon cancer? Studies have demonstrated that meat and dairy can be linked to cancer.(1) It turns out that what you eat is the single most potent weapon you have in the preventing disease and having a healthy life. With obesity rates and chronic illness increasing today more than ever and with our health care system now in jeopardy, the struggle for real, healthy food is not only important…it's critical for your brain and your moods.

So how do you begin?

Going vegan isn't for everyone. In fact, ditching meat can open the door to a bigger problem, such as emotional issues. If you live on cereals, chips, frozen vegan pizzas, store bought vegan cheeses, donuts, soy burgers, caffeine, bottled juices and soda, these can keep you in a fat, sick, and depressive stupor.

It's the simple steps you take every day that increases your health goals or sabotages them. Junk foods, fake foods, synthetic foods and processed chemical laden foods will always guarantee the making of a FAT VEGAN.

Choosing a healthy plan or making simple lifestyle changes means never going back to yo/yo dieting again. Great right? But, if you were 65+ pounds overweight when you began your plan to be healthier and 6 months later you're still 65+ pounds overweight, this book is for you. Please use this book as your toolkit for regaining your wellpower. Recovery from being sick, tired, depressed and fat brings an inner sense of peace, self-awareness, self-reflexion and self-love in every step you take towards change. As always, be kind to yourself and listen to your body.

> 'Most often it takes a collision
> with something or someone
> or with a situation
> that forces you to shift
> the course you are on'
>
> Caroline Myss

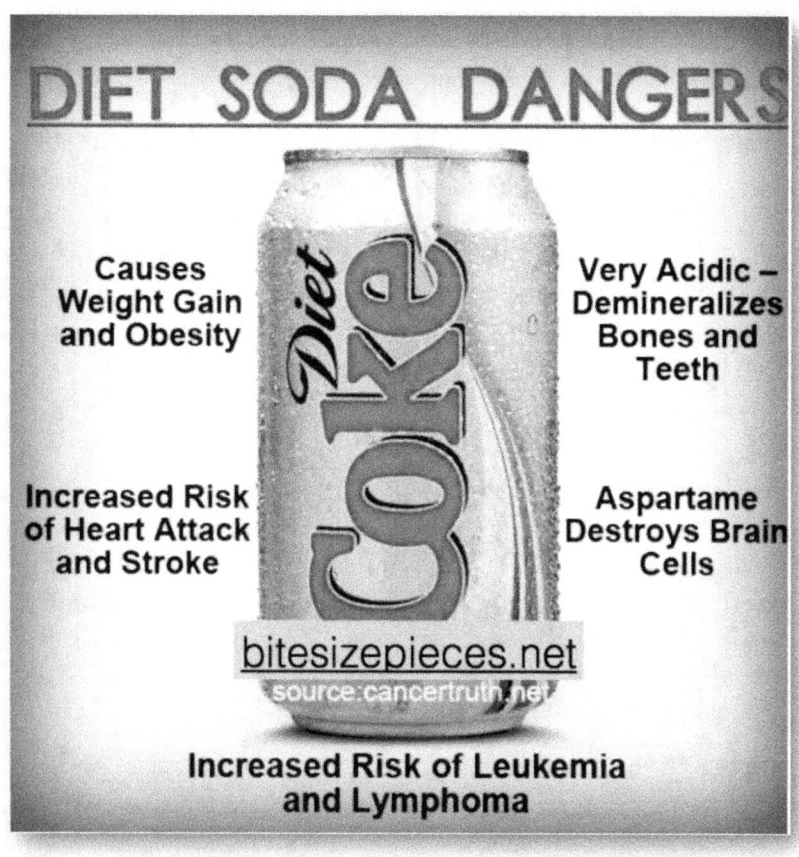

Zero Calories Makes a FAT VEGAN

Diet sugars are known to cause increased cravings, weight gain, brain toxicity and subsequently contribute to pre-diabetes.

To make matters worse, the synthetic estrogen, BPA can be found in your diet soda. Diet sodas can also contain the chemical and fake GMO sugar-substitute aspartame. You can't seem to pull yourself away from it because of it's addictive qualities. This kind of addiction causes a FAT VEGAN. In my research I've found there are over 92 different health side effects associated with aspartame consumption. One is aspartame decreases energy levels. See aspartame side effects on SweetPoison.com

Chemicals in diet sodas are just like drugs that can inhibit the production of vitamin B12, B6 and folate, when this happens the body has difficulty regulating other functions. This issue leads to an increased risk of cardiovascular disease. A lack of Vitamin B12 in the body is not from becoming vegan. Vitamin B12 is a bacteria, produced from microorganisms and is excreted in the bile and reabsorbed into the body.(2) A healthy digestive system and healthy liver is the key for healthy vitamin B12 levels in the body.

BPA's can also be found in canned foods. These disrupt our hormones and have been linked to serious health problems such as early puberty, and breast cancer. (3)

Diet By Numbers?

200 Calories From A Green Drink

Is Healthier than Zero Calories From Diet Sodas

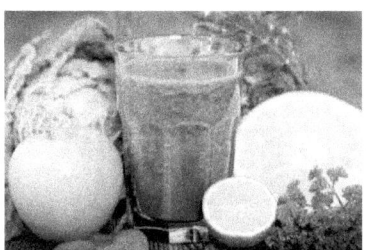
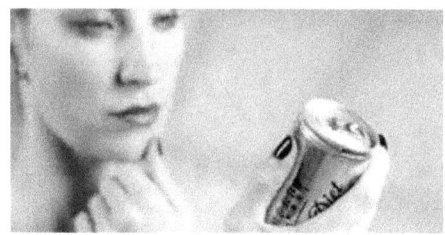

Simple Steps: It may be time to step into your pantry and remove old toxic canned foods and anything containing aspartame. Introduce organic seaweed, shitake mushrooms and parsley into your diet.

Avoid replacing diet soda with regular soda. Drinking regular cola increases ectopic fat accumulation and concentrations of triglycerides and total cholesterol compared with other drinks.(20) HFCS found in soda causes visceral fat.(22) This also increases your risk towards becoming a FAT VEGAN.

Eat at least 20% raw foods at every meal. You can start with a green smoothie in the am. Recipe found on page 49.

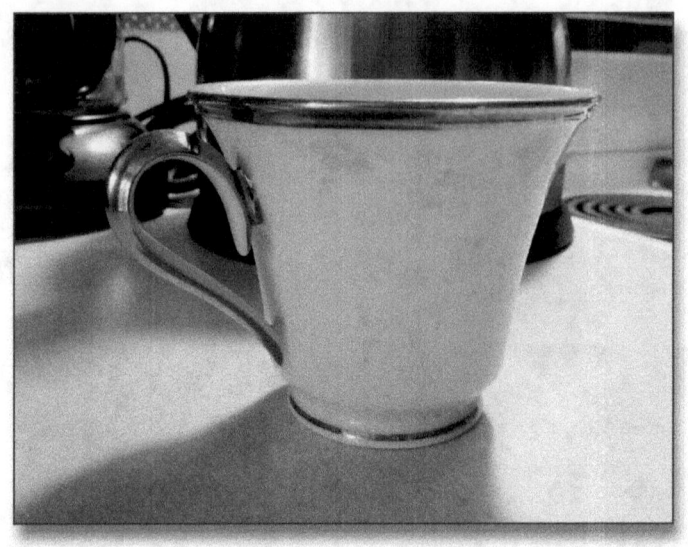

Your Morning Cup of Caffeine

Caffeine increases an acidic blood level and dehydration within the brain and body. A high caffeine diet depletes B vitamins and contributes to overeating. Studies tell us an abundance of caffeine in your day leads to insulin resistance and fat storage. This makes a Fat VEGAN

There is a myth that green tea is good for health. Green tea does not have metabolic benefits as previously thought. The FDA finds that existing evidence does not support qualified health claims for green tea consumption. Any spike in metabolic rate will be merely a spike and not a permanent change. Green tea can contain fluoride.

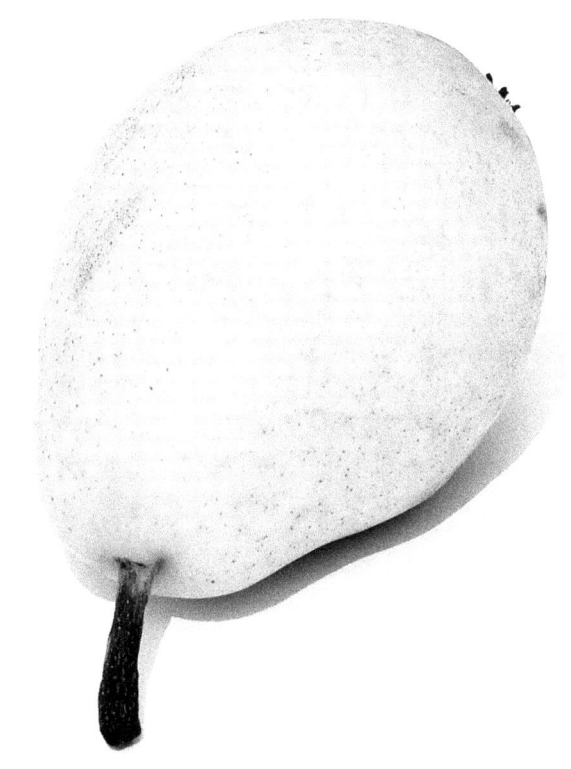

Vitamin C and Iron Absorption

"Iron Deficiency, according to the World Health Organization, is the number-one nutrition disorder in the world - affecting approximately 7.8 million women in the U.S. The most common symptoms of iron deficiency are fatigue, weakness, headaches and irritability." - (NewsUSA)

For vegans, some of us might be concerned about misinformation surrounding getting enough iron. And maybe you've heard of cereals, breads and pastas being advertised as, "iron fortified" or "iron enriched" whole grains? Crap!…You can't denature foods and then force synthetic vitamins in them and call them healthy. That's not how the body gets iron. The type of iron added to these isn't really a nutrient at all, but is considered a metallic iron. Metallic iron is not bioavailable to the human body and was never meant to be consumed.

Dried beans, lentils and dark green leafy vegetables such as kale and spinach and even tahini, (tahini inside hummus recipe at the end of this book) are especially good sources of iron, even better on a per calorie basis than meat. Not that we're counting calories!

Iron absorption is increased markedly by eating foods naturally high in vitamin C like pears and lemons, along with foods containing iron. Many vegetables such as broccoli and bok choy, which are high in iron, are also high in vitamin C so that the iron in these foods is very well absorbed. Vegans do not have a higher incidence of iron deficiency than do meat eaters, if they eat more veggies then they do sugar. An added bonus to being a vegan is nowadays more antibiotics are given to animals that are consumed than are distributed to people, which means that a lot of people are getting these drugs second-hand eating meat.

Simple Steps: When faced with misinformation research your choices.

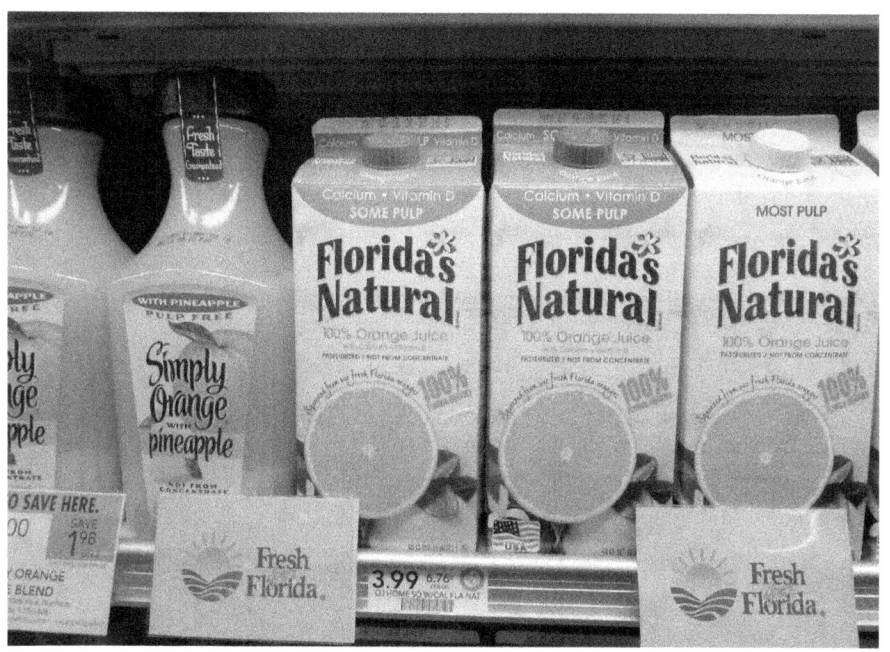

Your Orange Juice has been Hijacked

Adapted from My Natural News blog http://blogs.naturalnews.com/orange-juice-hijacked/

In the 1980's Tropicana coined the phrase "not from concentrate" to distinguish pasteurized orange juice from the "reconstituted concentrate brand". The idea was to convince us that pasteurized is a fresher, overall better product and so it cost more.(4) To make a product like orange juice taste fresh, chemicals have to be added. So to convince the masses, corporations put tons of advertising behind a product campaign and the result is an obese nation.

 Liquid sugar, is a term used for boxed, bottled, and canned juices. Liquid sugar is the single largest source of added sugar in the American diet.(5) Liquid sugar makes a FAT VEGAN and increases the risk for diabetes.

Everyday people can be confused with thousands of ad campaigns promoting mis-information in what's truly healthy and what's not, or what is fresh and what is not.

If you been deceived with fresh squeezed the solution is easier than you think.

Simple Steps: Choose foods that are living. Eat the whole organic orange and get all the fiber, vitamins and nutrients your body needs.

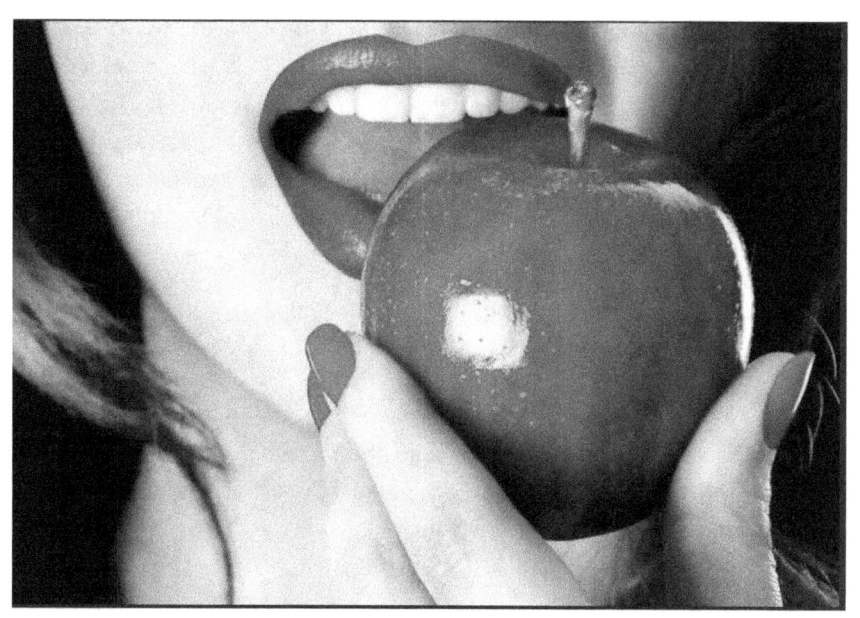

Do I Need Protein Substitutes?

The number one question that comes up in my coaching sessions is, "am I getting enough protein?" Followed by - "Do plants really have protein?" The answer is yes![1] Interestingly enough, three experts come to mind on this unique and controversial subject. According to Brian Clement at Hippocrates Institute in Florida, "wheatgrass (a superfood) contain over seventeen amino acids, which are the building blocks of protein and sprouted mung beans aren't far behind. It's a fact even athletes can get enough protein with plant based vegan food choices.

According to Dr. Fuhrman -exercise not protein builds strength and a plant based diet actually alkalizes the body for optimal bone health.(6)

If you are experiencing pain and inflammation in your joints and bones, listen up, according Alan Goldhamer an osteopathic physician at the True North Health Center in Santa Rosa, California reports, animal protein and animal fat are the major dietary promoters of arthritic pain.

Here are a few sources of plant based proteins:

☆ One ounce of pumpkin seeds contains 9.35 grams of protein.
☆ One ounce raw organic almonds contains about 6.03 grams of protein.
☆ One cup of chopped broccoli contains about 5.7 grams of protein.
☆ Two cups cooked spinach has about 10.70 grams of protein.
☆ Hemp seeds and chia seeds are also complete proteins.

---

[1] http://wp.me/p1otL6-Kh

So what is that processed toxic fungus "crap" in your protein substitute?

Mycoprotein is textured vegetable protein that is produced from a fungus, which can cause adverse reactions in people who are sensitive to its allergen. They may say it is good for people with high blood sugar, this however has never been proven.

According to John Robbins -

"Mycoprotein derived from Fusarium venenatum is almost certainly gastrotoxic. The risk of its toxicity does not justify its continued use here in the United States."

"Quorn is a chicken and meat substitute that originated in England. It is made from a fungus which has been likened to mushrooms, but, in fact is mold. Mold-did you know you are eating mold? Quorn is brewed up in big vats in a fermentation process similar to production of yogurt or beer, mixed with egg whites, flavored and shaped into foods resembling hamburgers and chicken tenders".

If you've think it's become mind boggling finding real food among the fake, you're not alone. Many "blueberry products" on the market today, contain no blueberries at all. Kellogg's™ "Blueberry Muffin" Frosted Mini Wheats cereal, for example, contains sugar, artificial dyes and genetically engineered soybean oil, but not a single blueberry. The same is true for many other foods being eaten by vegans every day. Blueberry muffins, bagels and pastries by Kellogg's,™ Betty Crocker™ and General Mills™ all show blueberries on the box, but contain no fruit.

Artificial dyes derived from petroleum are found in thousands of foods. These dyes can be cause for alarm, especially to children.(7) We consume it in candies, colored beverages, cereals, sodas, snow cones, birthday cakes and more. Only you have the power to ditch these and become a healthy vegan.

The truth is, we've all have been tricked into exposing ourself to processed, toxic crap when we stray from whole foods. Don't disable the body's self-healing potential by falling for false advertising. Take a step to remove one toxin a day out of your life.

Mis-information from a processed cereal company is marketing weight loss. When we read the labels we will be able to decipher what is real food and what is not.

> Kellogg's™ crisp-what will you gain when you lose? A catchy marketing term.
>
> ENRICHED FLOUR (WHEAT FLOUR, NIACIN, REDUCED IRON, THIAMIN MONONITRATE [VITAMIN B1], RIBOFLAVIN [VITAMIN B2], FOLIC ACID), SUGAR, FRUCTOSE, GLYCEROL, VEGETABLE OIL (SOYBEAN, PALM, AND PALM KERNEL OIL WITH TBHQ FOR FRESHNESS), DEXTROSE, MALTODEXTRIN, CONTAINS TWO PERCENT OR LESS OF MODIFIED CORN STARCH, NONFAT DRY MILK, APPLE POWDER, STRAWBERRY PUREE CONCENTRATE, REDUCED MINERAL WHEY, INVERT SUGAR, CORNSTARCH, SOY LECITHIN, LEAVENING (BAKING SODA, MONOCALCIUM PHOSPHATE, SODIUM ACID PYROPHOSPHATE), SALT, DATEM , CELLULOSE GEL, NATURAL AND ARTIFICIAL FLAVOR, CITRIC ACID, MONO- AND DIGLYCERIDES, CELLULOSE GUM, SODIUM CITRATE, MALIC ACID, COLOR ADDED, SODIUM ALGINATE, CARAMEL COLOR, XANTHAN GUM, TRICALCIUM PHOSPHATE, RED #40, VANILLA EXTRACT, BHT FOR FRESHNESS.

Simple Steps: Make your breakfast enjoyable and creative. Don't believe a processed cereal such as Cheerios can contain all the protein you need.(21) Hemp seed protein and hemp hearts is the best protein you can put in your smoothie, or you can make your own cereal with it and leave the boxed cereal behind forever.

My Favorite Home Made Organic Cereal Recipe

1/2 cup organic buckwheat groats
1/4 cup raw organic pumpkin seeds
1/4 cup raw organic hemp hearts
2 Tablespoons organic chia seeds
2 Tablespoons organic shredded unsweetened coconut
1 Tablespoon organic ground cinnamon

Combine ingredients and place in sealed container and use 1/4 cup of this mixture for breakfast. Optional- top with 1/4 cup of organic berries.

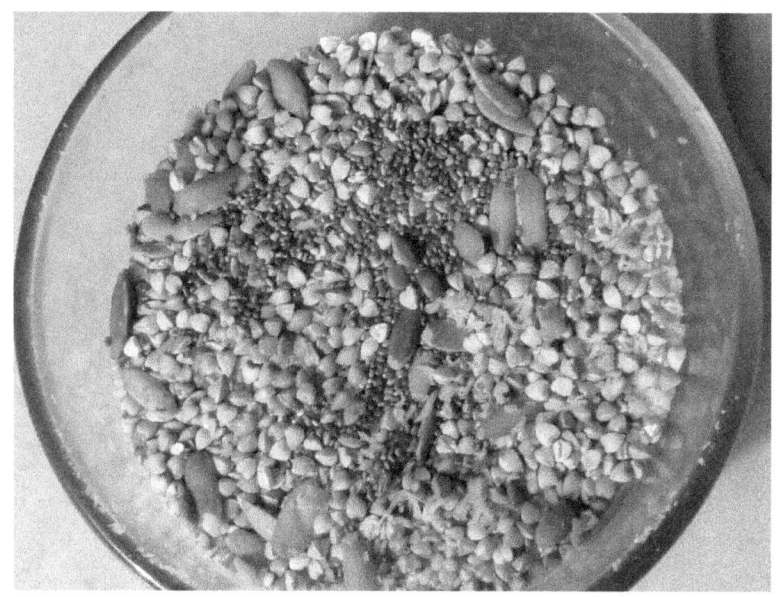

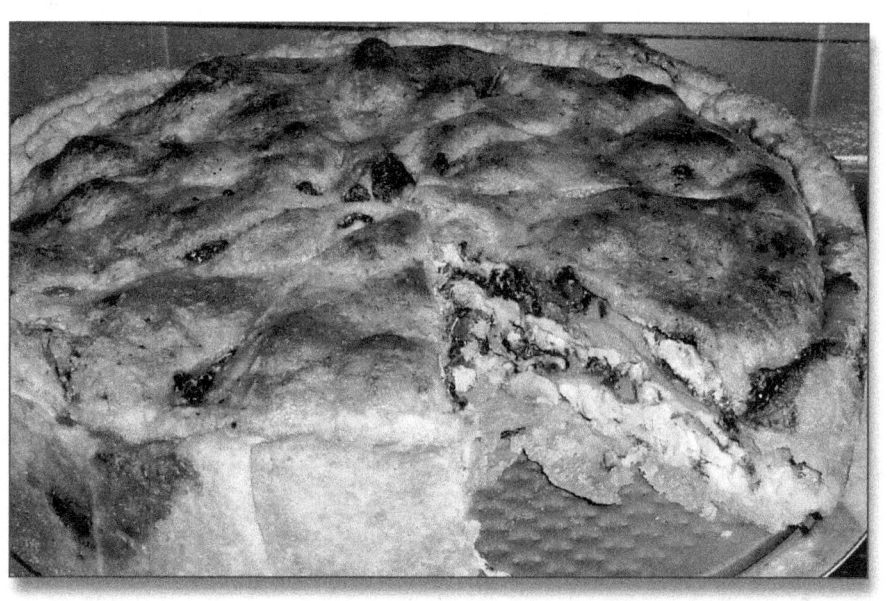

Wheat is not The Staff of Life

Research claims there are no nutritional differences between organic wheat and non-organic wheat, according to a 2006 article published in the Journal of Agricultural & Food Chemistry.

Really?

So what about those toxins, pesticides and "crap" hormones on wheat? According to Dr. Mercola, "Many forget that most commercial wheat production is, unfortunately, a study in pesticide application, beginning with the seeds being treated with fungicide."

Once seeds become wheat, they are sprayed with hormones and pesticides. Sounds strange, but farmers apply hormone-like substances or "plant growth regulators" that affect wheat characteristics, time of germination and strength of stalk. Cycocel is a synthetic hormone that is commonly applied to wheat. Eating these foods is more likely to cause a gluten allergy and in fact can increase your risk of getting cancer.(8) These chemicals all contribute to increasing the average person's toxic load, which is a contributing factor to virtually every possible disease imaginable.

Products that advertise themselves as "100% whole wheat" are legally required to be just that. But there is currently no definition on the percentage of "whole wheat" required to advertise a product as "made with whole wheat." In many cases manufacturers will incorporate a small amount of whole wheat and then add caramel color to white flour-filled "crap" products, knowing consumers will fall for the dark look and the "made with whole wheat" claim.

Ditch Soups with Dry Packaged Noodles

Instant noodle products are a processed food and made to withstand a long shelf life. This means they can contain, artificial colors, dyes, chemicals, trans-fats, dirty toxic salt, preservatives and flavorings. These flavorings can be high in MSG, an excitotoxin, that makes you want to eat more, causing a FAT VEGAN.

"Women who ate instant noodles twice a week or more had a higher risk of metabolic syndrome than those who ate less, or not at all, regardless of whether their diet style fell into the traditional or fast-food category, " as published in *The Washington Post*

Simple Steps: Bread or instant noodles should never be considered a healthy or even a necessary part of the diet.

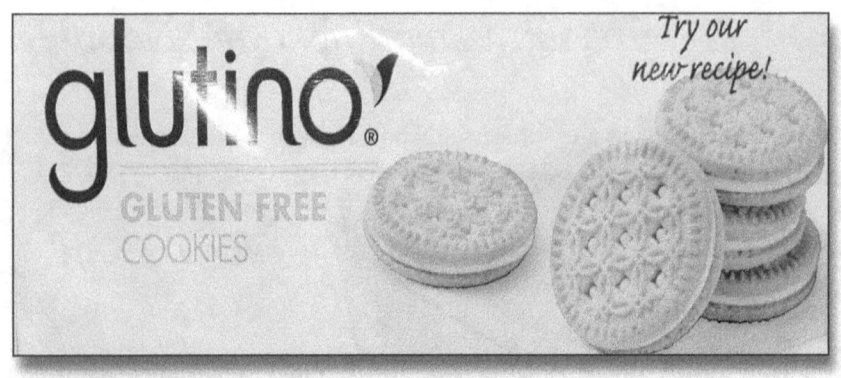

Don't Get Caught Buying Gluten-free

As of 2014, the FDA finalize the regulation defining gluten-free. (13) The FDA states that labeling a food as gluten-free is acceptable as long as it is truthful and not misleading. Without testing levels of gluten, it's possible that foods containing higher than 20 ppm gluten could be labeled gluten-free and purchased by unsuspecting consumers. A 2010 study found that gluten-free flours, such as rice and soy, can contain significant levels of gluten, raises a concern about the content of gluten in flours that food manufacturers are using for gluten-free products." (14) Additionally gluten-free products can contain Synthetics, GMO's and MSG ingredients.

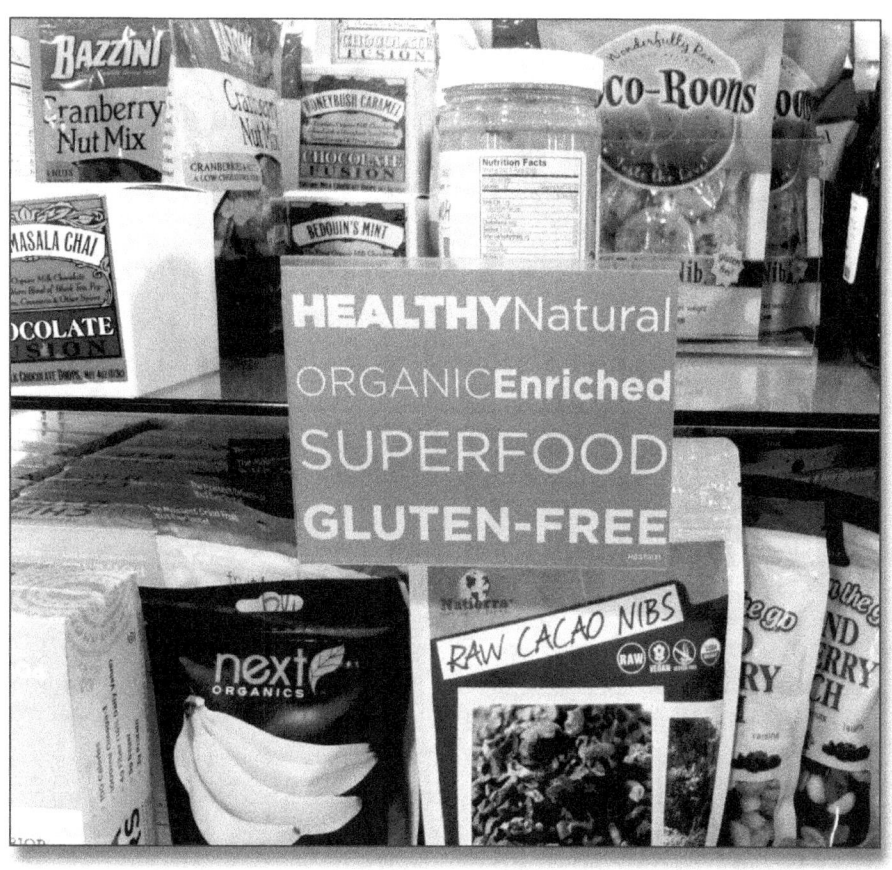

Natural Isn't Natural

"All Natural" is just a marketing ploy... period.

The words- Natural, Smart, Gluten-Free and Conventional - do not necessarily mean they are good for our health. Contrary to popular belief these words can actually mean chemicals, synthetics, toxins and pesticides in both food & skin care products. Environmental chemicals known as *obesogens* are found in many places, including pesticides used on conventional produce. They program our bodies to store fat and develop disease.

Today, foods that are called "natural" or contain natural flavors are used to trick us into thinking they're good for us. They are made in a way that makes them palatable. Examples are found in soda's, growth hormones in wheat, chemicals in orange juice, genetically engineered corn in corn flakes, and caramel coloring in processed foods and drinks are just a few examples. Caramel coloring has been proven to increase risk of obesity and cancer. (9) Some juices can even contain levels of arsenic and lead.(10)

Have you been tricked by"slimsweet"? One customer did his own research... He said "I've been searching ....for a "luo han sweetener" to alleviate my blood sugar problems. Unfortunately, I was duped by this product. The ingredients list "levulose" as well as the lo han content (a "proprietary blend" of the two). Levulose, he discovered upon investigation, is refined fructose. Nice ploy to make it look like something else."

All these tricks can add to the making of a FAT VEGAN.

Simple Steps: When choosing organic vs. a regular conventional product there is nothing conventional about it. If the signs in the grocery store said, laden with several harmful pesticides, resins, synthetics and hormones, OR this is a genetically modified food, would you think differently?

Let me say this, there is so much more healthy food choices you can eat to feed your mind and body. Unless you eat from Mother Natures Table you are not doing a body good.

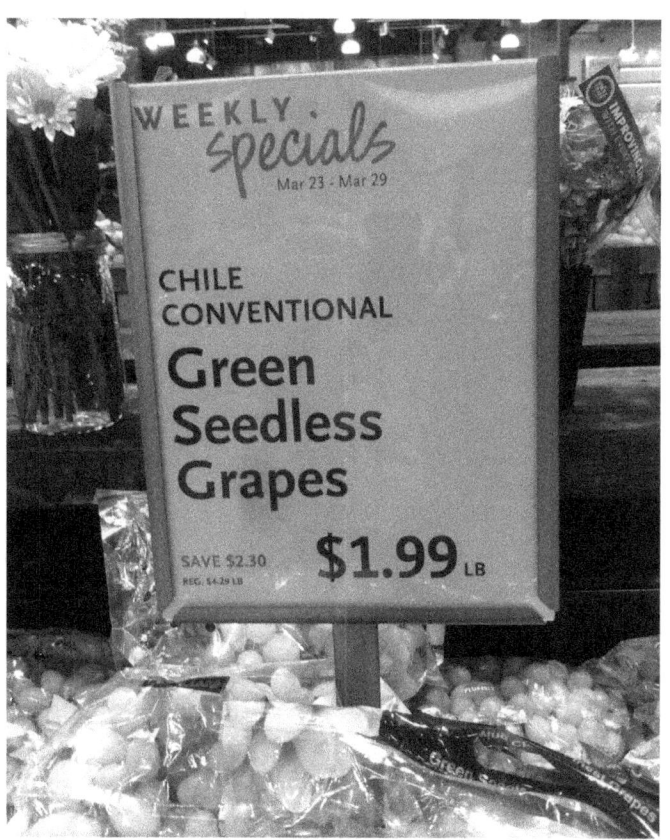

Don't be fooled by conventional

Here are some sites where Corporations have been SUED for calling their products natural.

B&G foods lawsuit for misleading shoppers on all natural claim. http://mobile.foodnavigator-usa.com/Regulation/B-G-Foods-hit-with-natural-lawsuit-over-artificial-ingredients-GMOs#.VE_Q-r62-zd

General Mills loses lawsuit on saying their products are Natural. https://www.organicconsumers.org/news/general-mills-agrees-drop-"100-natural"-labeling-face-lawsuit

ConAgra GMO Wesson oil is not Natural. http://www.treehugger.com/corporate-responsibility/conagra-sued-for-misusing-100-natural-claim-on-genetically-modified-oils.html

Frito Lay is not Natural. http://www.treehugger.com/corporate-responsibility/frito-lay-sued-for-labeling-gmo-ingredients-as-all-natural.html

We live in a system that doesn't honor what nature's all about. (11)

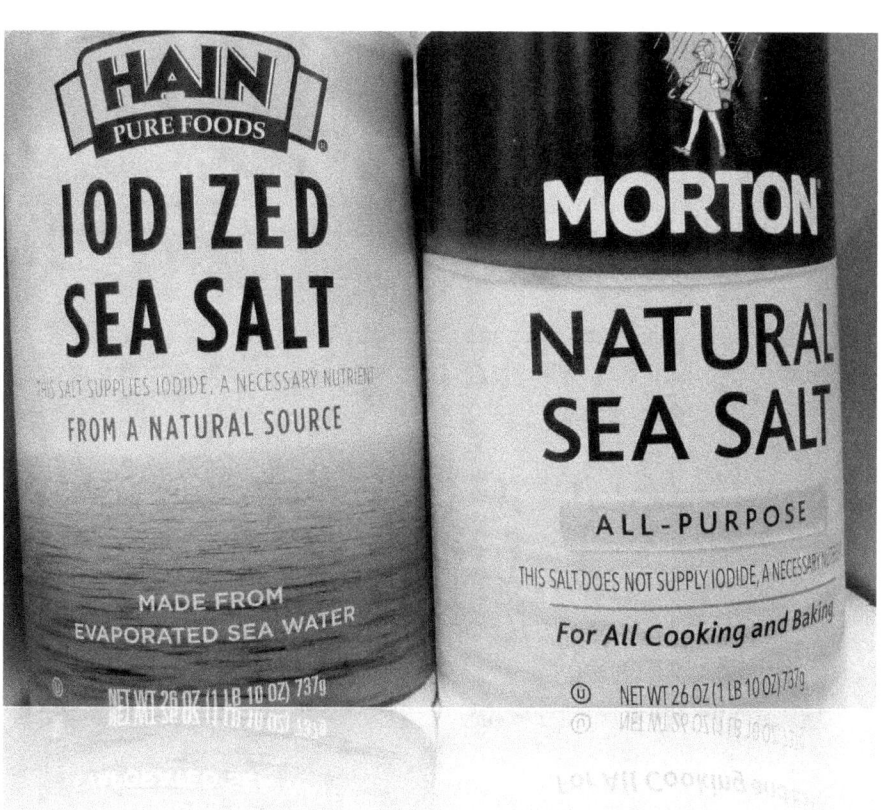

The Scoop on Toxic Salts

Most Restaurants, boxed and frozen foods are packed with toxic dirty salts that have been bleached and denatured. Almost 80% of these dirty salts we consume are found in processed foods we buy such as chips, protein bars, candy, marinades, ketchup, canned soups, instant noodles, fries, desserts, roasted nuts, peanut butters and more. These are the salts that add to a FAT VEGAN.

An example is morning star frozen breakfast patties, which contain toxic denatured salts, chemical laden eggs, trans-fats, toxic vegetable oils, iron, food coloring, MSG, (sugars listed 5 times), wheat-gluten and GMO soy, milk, corn and corn sugar ingredients.

Moving on.. we may find ourselves eating and drinking toxic salt ingredients in our canned soups and electrolyte products such as gatorade.

The body needs good salts.

- ☆ Our body needs salt to survive.
- ☆ Sweat is salt!
- ☆ Salt regulates blood sugar.
- ☆ Without salt- we'd develop confusion and altered mental states, fatigue and edema/dropsy, just to name a few.
- ☆ We need salt to avoid dehydration.

Organic Dulse granules comes from seaweed. It has the nutritional benefits of sea vegetables. This seaweed grows in the cold waters of the North Atlantic Ocean on rocks at the low tide line where currents are strong and the bottom is clean.

Simple Steps: Ditch those toxic bleached salts that pretend to be good salts. You can purchase non-toxic grey celtic sea salt or dulse granules.

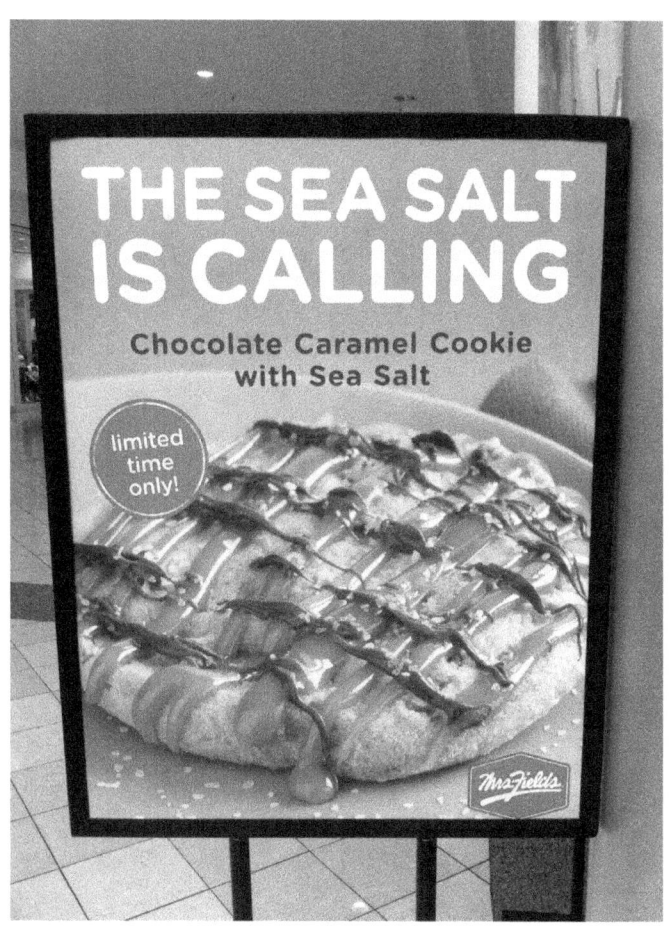

Visual temptation with misinformation

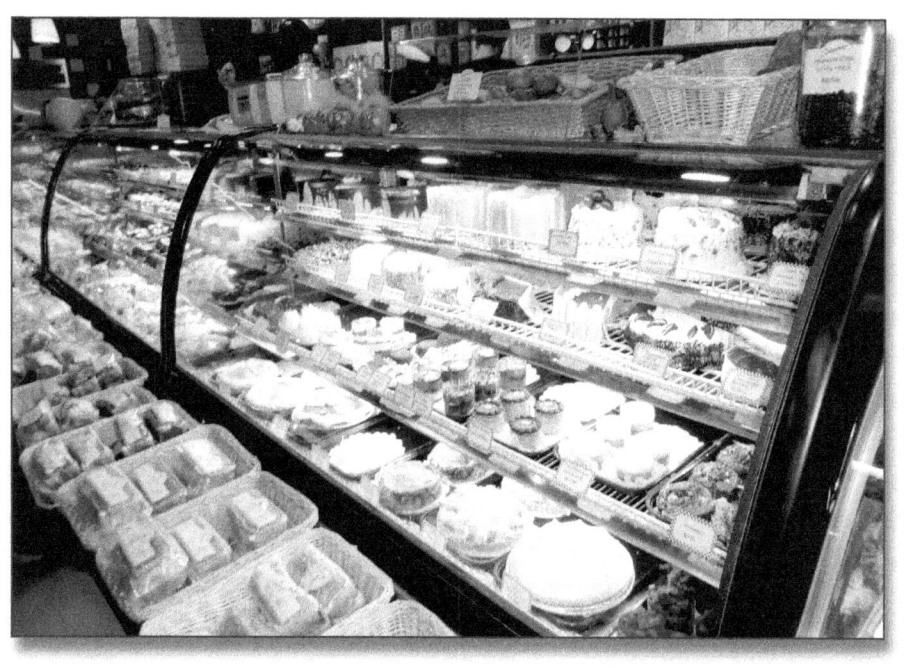

Let's Talk GMO's

Have you seen maltodextrin and dextrose on the labels of your favorite foods? GMO bacteria and fungi are used in the production of enzymes, vitamins, food additives, flavorings and processing agents in thousands of foods on the grocery shelves as well as health supplements. Peppers for instance, are sprayed over 700 times with pesticides. Most packaged foods contain GMO soy and/or corn in some form, such as soy flour, soy protein, soy lecithin, textured vegetable protein, corn meal, corn syrup, dextrose, maltodextrin, fructose, citric acid, lactic acid, and of course, soy or corn oil. So if we just single out corn for example, it encourages weight gain by disrupting gut bacteria. This includes popcorn. Popcorn is not a health food or a healthy snack. Nutrient levels are depleted while obesity rises, making you a FAT VEGAN.

So, how do you protect your family from fake food?

Simple Steps: Reading ingredient labels is the first step. If your snacks consist of BT (GMO) corn chips, crackers, peanut butter and beer, you can make the decision to make healthier choices. Yes even peanut butter is not a healthy food, because of it's moldy content and unwanted metabolic side effects. This mold produces aflatoxins that can harm our mind and body. Peanut butter ingredients can also contain toxic salts and vegetable oils, making you a FAT VEGAN.

It's important to know what you're eating. Ask-Is it real or processed? You can make organic raw almond butter in the comfort of your home using your Blendtec.

Know your food, and know your farmer.

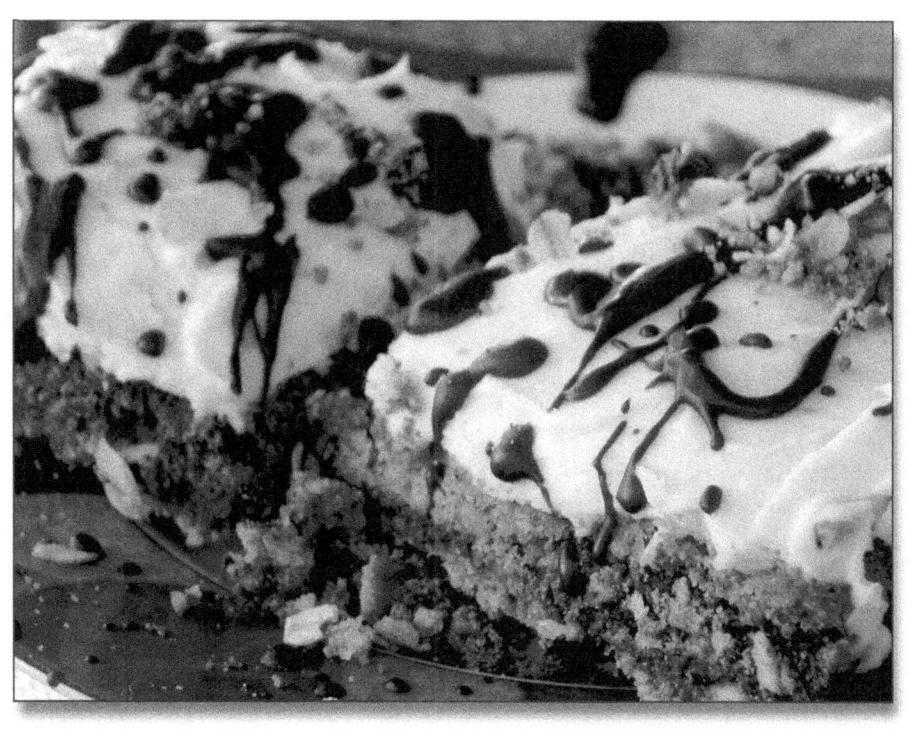

Sugar Equals a FAT VEGAN

Big Corporations need us to buy their stuff even if it cost us our lives. Is it acceptable to eat a ton of sugar just because you're vegan?

Unfortunately Belly Fat equal estrogen dominance. In the "buffet of life" there are certain things we do every day not knowing the impact it may have on our health, such as chronic dieting. Loosing weight and gaining weight over and over again is not good for our health or weight loss efforts. A lack of oxygen rich foods and an oxygen poor lifestyle can add more fat in the belly. Before you know it you can become riddled with stress, confusion, fat and undesirable health challenges.

It can be important to know the reason for our "estrogen" excess.Fact: High Estrogen levels means the mind can have problems concentrating, as estrogen affects cognitive function and our moods.(12) When this happens, we become lethargic, depressed and fat.

Poor nutrition equals more belly fat. Fat cells store toxins and here's why… Adipose tissue is not simply an inert storage depot for lipids but is also an important endocrine organ."(15) When we gain belly-fat the body is toxic.

I have seen so many athletes eating a sugary breakfast before an intense workout, and experiencing heart troubles on the court. The crash is not fun, and could be life threatening. Years ago, I was invited to be part of a 60 mile bike race in Temecula California. There, I witnessed what athletes ate for breakfast, and it wasn't pretty. They consumed tons of caffeine, donuts, rice cakes and sugary products. I call this the useless food group, because they do nothing but spike blood sugar levels. In the evening of this event when all was said and done, alcohol was their game. If you are consuming sugary foods and drinking alcohol you are setting yourself up to be a FAT VEGAN. Refined sugar is a drug and causes all kinds of digestive issues along with inflammation and depression. It's a set up for moods disorders, insulin resistance, hormonal imbalances and disease.

The good news is, when blood sugar levels are balanced, we crave less sugar.

When you are adding nutritious foods into your body, you are on the right tract to making a healthy vegan.

Being vegan for whatever your reason, is an investment in yourself. Eating junk and sugar is counterproductive.

Simple Step for less belly fat: Cruciferous vegetables can be eaten for lunch or dinner and they fight belly fat. In fact, these healthy foods can improve your mood and weight.

Metabolic Disruption

Metabolic Disruption includes Insulin Resistance, Diabetes, Cancer, Heart Disease, Obesity, Hypoglycemia and Thyroid disorders.

If we just single out the thyroid we will find children are developing more thyroid disorders at an earlier age. Thyroid disorders can be linked not only to a relationship with an abundance of sugar, but also with fluorides found in our diet. Facts are, fluoride can increase insulin resistance.[2]

The thyroid gland is central to the regulation of our metabolism. So if the thyroid is not functioning properly, every other organ system in the body starts malfunctioning. Fluoride can affect the gut in a negative fashion. Our gut microbiome influences our weight, immunity and insulin levels and therefore plays a role in all autoimmunity disorders. When connecting the dots we can safely say there is a direct connection from ingestion of fluorides and a FAT VEGAN.

Simple Steps: Get a water filter that clears out the fluoride and chlorine.

---

[2] http://fluoridealert.org/studies/diabetes02/

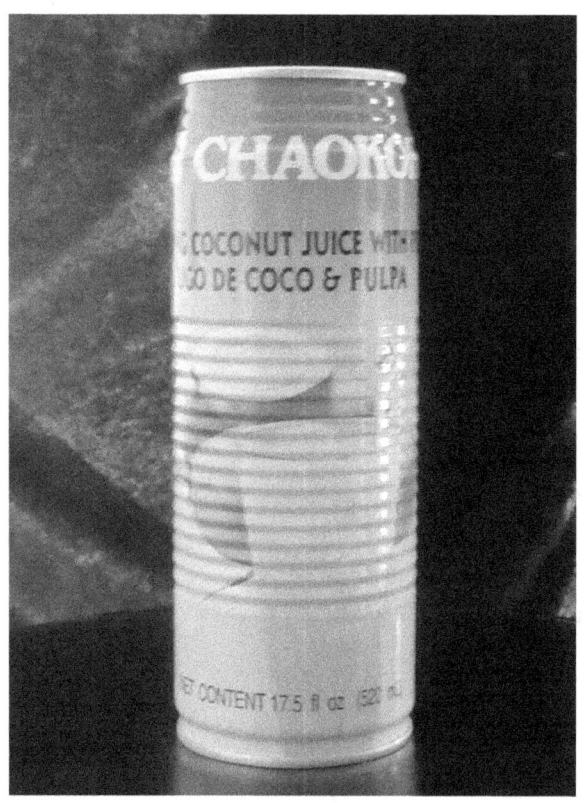

Are you tricked into thinking this is water?

Hydration for Life!

We can't survive too many days without drinking pure clean water. Water assist the body in flushing out waste while all elimination systems work more effectively. In fact, there are times when you think you're hungry but if you just take the time to drink a glass of water that may satisfy your cravings. Best bet is to keep a glass water bottle or stainless steel water bottle with you at all times.

While many think coconut waters are healthy and natural, they are not. The best healthy coconut water is directly from the coconut. Canned coconut water may contain unnatural flavors, synthetic vitamins, GMO sugars, and may be packaged in leaching aluminum cans.

Simple Steps: Make sure you drink plenty of good clean water daily. Being hydrated increases energy levels.

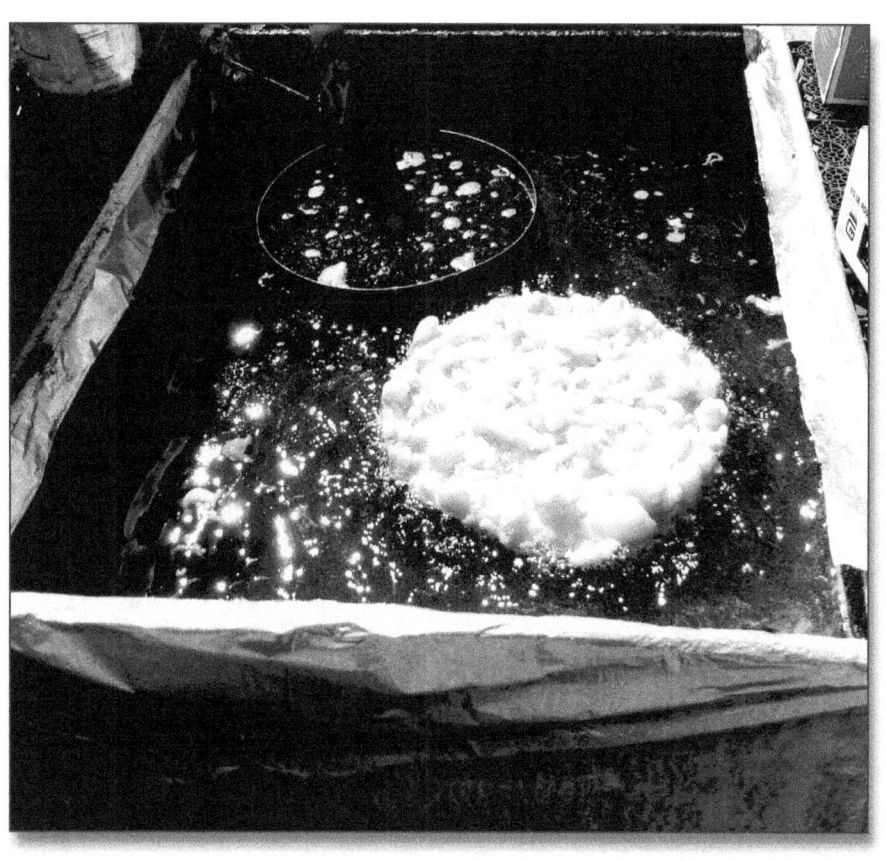

Fat Facts

Advertisers have us fearing fat as though it were poison, when the truth is all fats are not your enemy.

Fat-free foods can trick us into believing they don't cause fat gain, when in fact they do. Fat-free can be loaded with sugars.

Trans-fats are toxic fats. These can be found in vegetable oils, microwaved popcorn, roasted nuts, salad dressings, pie crust, deep fried foods, margarine, canned frosting, non-dairy creamers and much more.

Trans-fats promote heart disease as well as diabetes and are toxic to our brain. They are used to extend a product's shelf life. Trans-fats are suppose to be labeled, but there's a loophole, where they can list canola and soy oil instead.

Vegetable oils are oils chemically extracted from seeds like sunflower and other oils. They are processed, deodorized, and altered. These are some of the most chemically dangerous foods in our diets and some are even promoted as healthy.

Simple Steps: Add good fats into your diet such as organic raw almonds, organic unrefined cold pressed coconut oil and avocado's. Delete toxic vegetable oils and roasted nuts. Eat to remove belly fat.[3]

---

[3] blogs.naturalnews.com/eat-remove-belly-fat/

The Salad Dressing Addiction

Spring season is prime time for big colorful salads, especially when you add fresh basil, tomatoes and bell peppers from your garden. How do you spell fresh? Or, how about visiting your local farmers markets that just picked their fresh organic produce at 5 am and you are there by 9 am.

I love the taste and smell of a great salad sprinkled with a little fresh lemon and a few herbs. Yum. However, I have found many of my clients and friends like to bury their masterpiece by overdressing it. Yes, they dump a toxic goo like substance on top of a big beautiful fresh, organic, salad and call it a dressing. Yuck!

If you one of those that can't have salad without your favorite store bought bottled dressing, than you may be addicted.(16)

Adding a chemical laden store-bought salad dressing into the equation, changes the goodness of your intentions and your salad. Most store bought salad dressings are anything but fresh. They are filled with hard to pronounce chemicals and other "unnecessary" toxic ingredients such as HFCS and titanium dioxide.

I have read salad dressing labels that contain fifteen or more toxins that we don't need in our body, making it increasingly difficult to digest. The repercussions can keep us in a state of addiction and IBS. Corporate advertising wants us to believe trans-fats, dirty salts, GMO cornstarch, GMO sugars, fake flavors, MSG, excitotoxins, synthetics and colors are foods that are yummy and/or healthy. They disguise the taste of these false and dangerous flavors engineered in a laboratory. These synthetics are toxic to our lymph, colon and immune system. Salad dressings can lead to a FAT VEGAN.

Simple Steps: Make your own salad dressing or buy raw salad dressings.

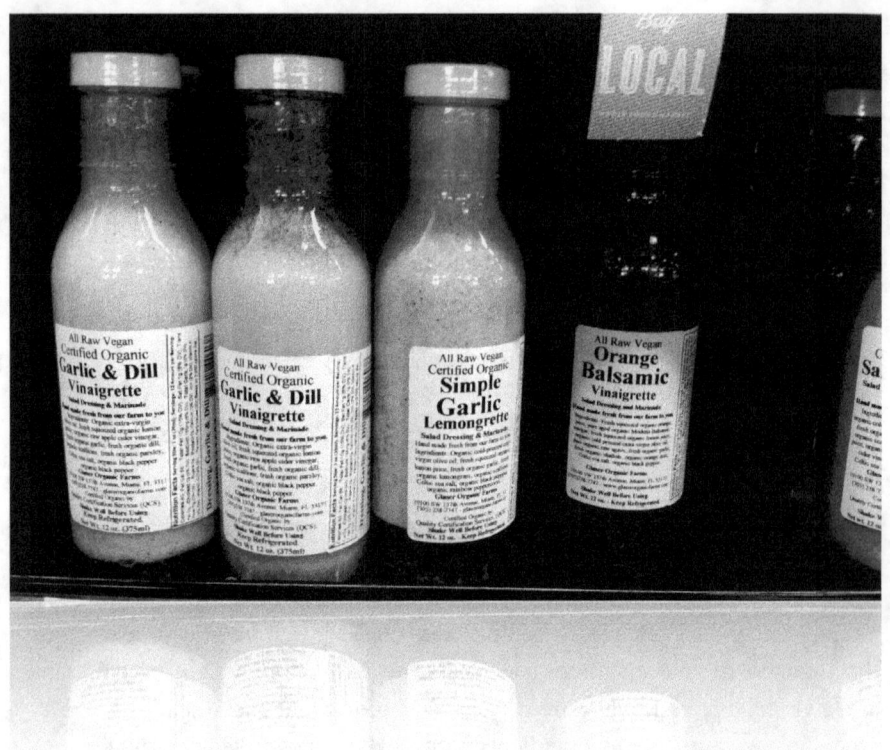

Raw Organic Salad Dressing

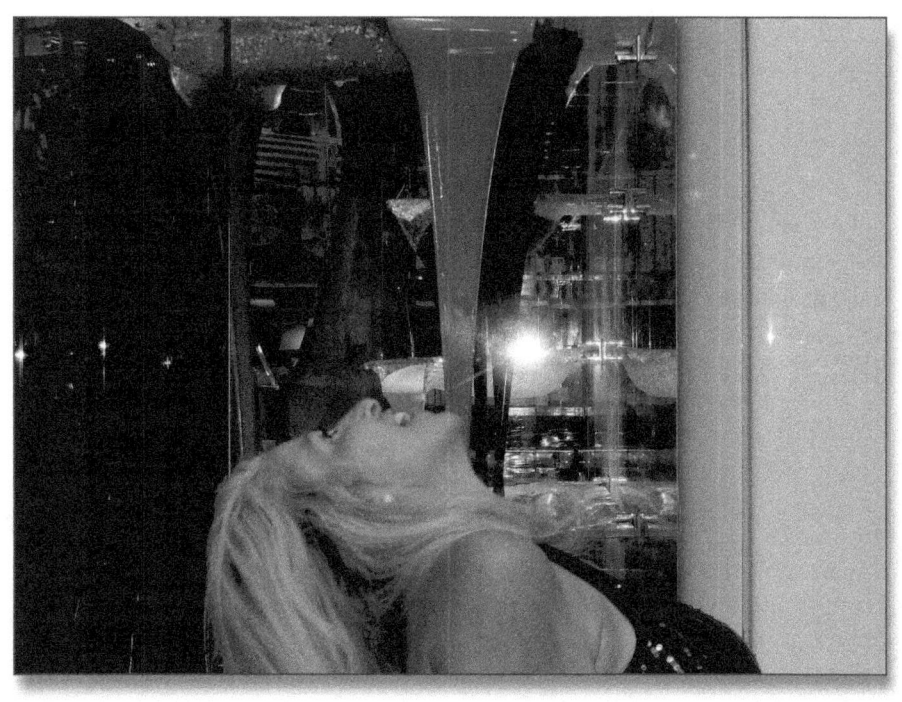

Your Mental Muscle

Being stressed weakens your mental muscle. Insomnia can be one example of our body's response to an abundance of stress. The body naturally releases toxins, rebuilds and rejuvenates when we sleep. Lack of sleep can keep us sick and make us a FAT VEGAN.

If we experience inflammation in our body it is also in our brain. Our gut and brain work in tandem, each influencing the other. Chemicals and synthetics in our food play a causative role in inflammation which disrupts our cholesterol, blood sugar and cortisol levels and appears to significantly increase the risk of dementia, Alzheimer's, diabetes, heart disease and weight gain.

This leads to the question, have you been tricked into eating synthetic food? Hell, China's making plastic and cardboard food products and people are eating them. (19) Corporations think that synthetics are the way to feed the world hunger crisis. And they are finding ways to put synthetics into vegan based foods.(17) It's never a good idea to eat these synthetic fake-meat products.

Synthetic toxins can disrupt hormones and increase our stress levels, disrupt our brain function all the while increasing obesity. Fact: Dr Daniel Amen says, "Obese people have smaller brains." This is when size matters most!

Simple Steps: Explore and overcome sources of resistances and remind yourself of the benefits of moving past them. Embrace change. Incorporate better sleeping habits.

Emotions

It's well known that emotions and stress can cause a FAT VEGAN and other disorders. So the question is: Do people just have weight issues because of imbalances in metabolism or can they be repressing depressive memories? For instance, if you were abused sexually, your body can also have issues with metabolism imbalances. Your body keeps SCORE. (Single Concentration Of Repressed Emotions) If consciousness is blocked you can years later experience blockages in other parts of the body.

Simple Steps: Today more than ever there are resources available so you don't have to continue suffering. You can make simple, yet powerful lifestyle changes that can release buried emotional stress. You can choose to remain with people that love you and release toxic relationships. You can work through your pain and increase your wellpower muscle with a Certified Health Coach.

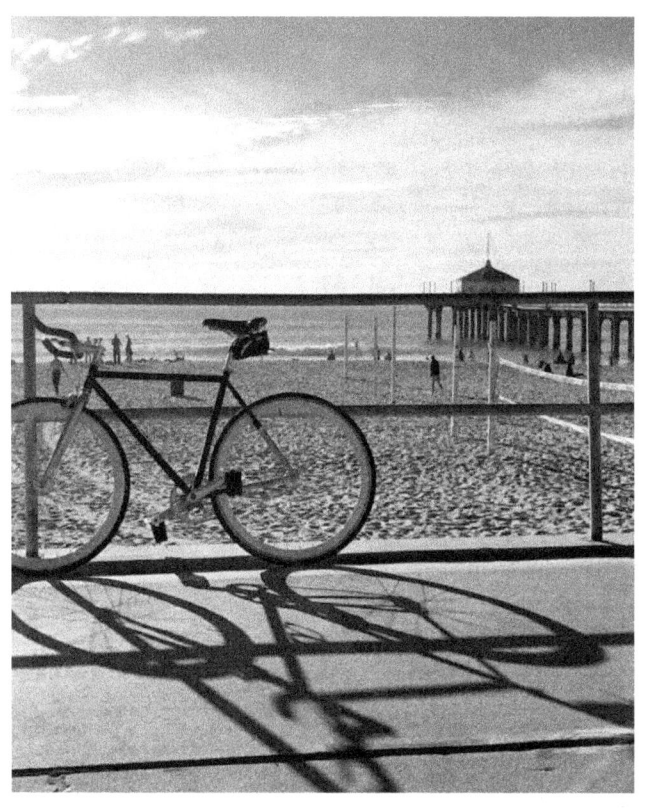

All Life is Movement

A sedentary lifestyle, such as watching TV after work can increase weight gain. The average person is receiving twelve hours a day of information overload. This can keep our brain and body from functioning optimally and lethargic. We thrive best when we keep moving. It's a good idea to make a commitment to ourselves to include daily exercise and self-care habits.

All life is movement includes every cell in the body eliminating toxic waste. This means we need to poop like a rock star and not ever poop rocks! If we aren't moving our bowels 2 times a day we are constipated. Daily bowel movements are important. We can even be constipated when we have loose bowels, leaky gut or diarrhea.(18) Allergies, mood disorders and poor digestive health can be signs of leaky gut. For your digestive health, leafy green veggies are the perfect food.(23)

Good elimination habits begin with chewing your food. Tasting food requires exciting all senses. What can you do? Sit down and relax when you eat.

The skin also eliminates toxic waste. We can assist the body with the elimination process by adding dry brushing to our morning routine and exercise to our day. Dry brushing and exercise are good for circulation, bone health, stimulation of the lymph glands and the digestive system.

Steps to a healthy elimination system is directly linked to getting a good nights sleep. So we can safely say: Eating, Moving and Sleeping are important for you to heal and thrive.

Simple Steps: When we make a decision for better health, it's a movement to insure results.

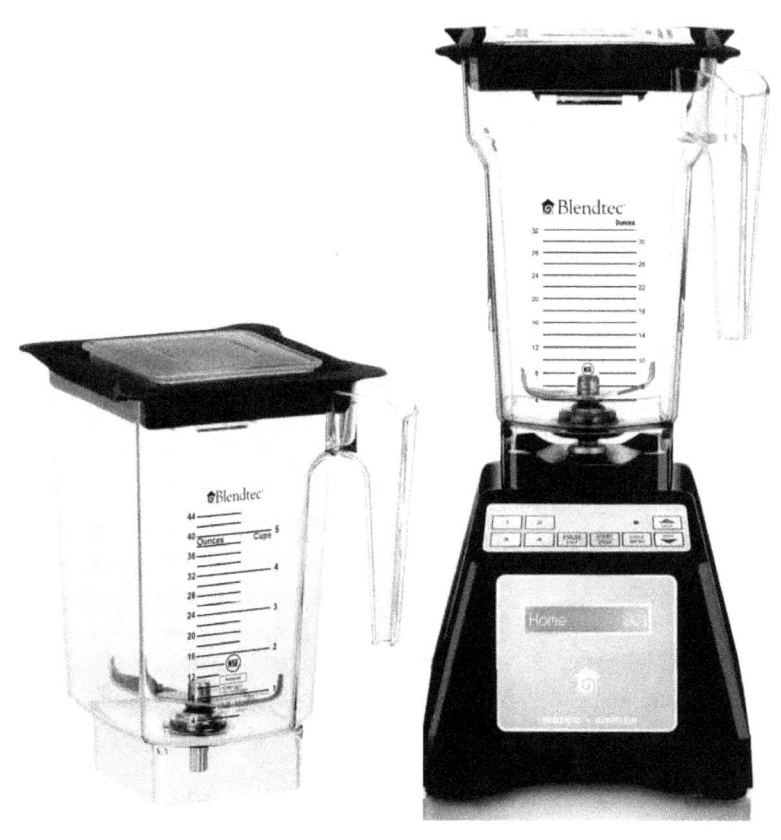

Kitchen Tools

You can jumpstart your metabolism. Metabolism is the process by which the body breaks down food and converts that food to energy. Food is the building blocks of energy. Fruits like pineapple help increase metabolism because of all the extra fibers they provide. The path to decreasing the prevalence of obesity, cancer, and illness is to change the way we look at our food. Eating meat no longer has the implications that we are wealthier or wiser than our neighbor next door. In fact, it could mean just the opposite.

Simple Steps: Start investing. If you would like to drink a delicious smoothie in the morning -invest in a Blendtec Blender. Learn why you need a Blentec in your kitchen [4]

If you would like to make your own flax seed crackers -invest in a dehydrator.

If you want to make your juices at home-invest in a juicer.

If you want to loose some extra pounds the only real way to change your weight, gain energy and feel better, is to change your mind. Then change the way you eat and exercise.

Remember: Deciding not to eat meat doesn't mean we have to be an outcast or ousted from the family fun. It's time to be kind and considerate to others special needs and/or choices.

---

[4] www.kqzyfj.com/click-7211658-11657061

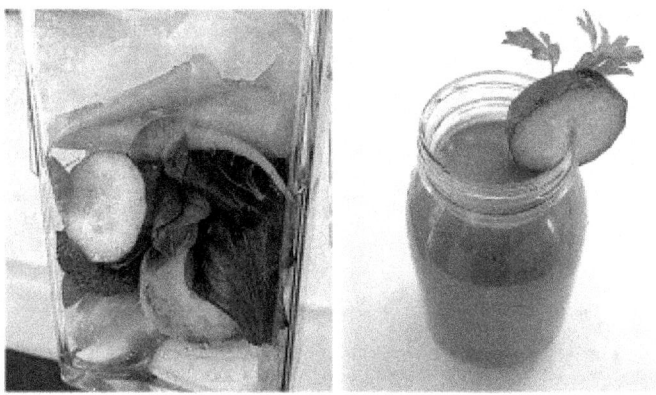

Green Sunshine Smoothie

3 organic large kale leaves (stems removed)
1/2 organic cucumber (quartered)
1 organic carrot
1 thumb size piece of organic ginger root
1 organic green apple (sliced)
1/2 organic banana
1/2 organic avocado (pitted)
1/4 cup raw organic cashews (optional)
1/4 cup organic hemp seeds
1 teaspoon fresh mint leaves
2 cups plain water
2 cups ice

Blend all ingredients together in your Blendtec to get desired consistency. Ridiculously Delicious!

Health Benefits below:

A super food for life – one cup of **Kale** contains vitamins K, A, C, B6, E plus minerals such as, manganese, copper, calcium, potassium, iron, and magnesium. Kale contains powerful antioxidants that protect our cells from free radicals that cause oxidative stress. The high fiber content of kale lowers our cholesterol by binding with bile acids that the liver produces from cholesterol for digesting fat.

Apples help you to wake up in the morning and are good for your brain power. Research has shown that people who eat fruits and other high-fibre foods gain a certain amount of protection against Parkinson's. Apples are considered a good source of immune system-boosting vitamin C. In 2004 WebMD reported, French research found that a chemical in apples helped prevent colon cancer. And in 2007, a study from Cornell University found additional compounds in apples called triterpenoids, which seem to fight against liver, colon, and breast cancers.

Ginger has been in use since ancient times for its anti-inflammatory, carminative, as well as anti-bacterial and anti-microbial properties.

Raw Cashews have a lower fat content than most other nuts and most of it is in the form of oleic acid. Studies show that oleic acid promotes good cardiovascular health by helping to reduce triglyceride levels. Raw cashews are particularly rich in magnesium.

Avocados are high in beta-sitosterol, a compound that has been shown to lower cholesterol levels. The high levels of folate in avocado are protective against strokes and heart disease.

Cucumbers are 95 percent water, keeping the body hydrated while helping the body eliminate toxins. Adding cucumbers to your routine is ideal for people who are looking for weight loss. Cucumbers are a good source of B vitamins.

Mint acts as a cooling sensation to the skin and helps in dealing with skin irritations. It helps in eliminating toxins from the body, aids in digestion and is a very good cleanser for the blood.

A serving of **Carrots** will provide 400% of your daily vitamin A, B1, B2, B3, B6, C, E and K, and plenty of fiber, manganese and potassium and can help to prevent heart disease and cancer, as well as protecting your vision. Carotenoids inversely affect insulin resistance and thus lower blood sugar.

Hemp seeds are the best protein for smoothies. According to a research study published in the journal "Bioscience, Biotechnology, and Biochemistry," hemp seeds are a complete protein, meaning they contain every essential amino acid.

Bananas are rich in vitamin B6 and are a good source of fibre, vitamin C, magnesium and potassium. Vitamin B6 helps prevent irritability and insomnia. Potassium helps regulate blood pressure and can also reduce the risk of high blood pressure and stroke. Potassium also prevents the bloods pH from becoming too acidic.

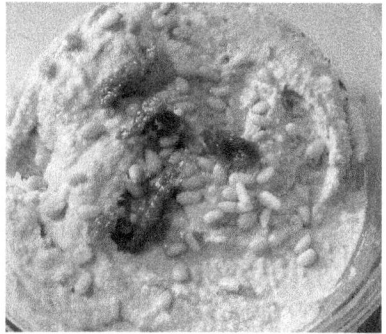

Hummus Recipe

One 15 oz can organic garbanzo beans (drained)
One small zucchini (peeled and chopped)
2 fresh lemons (juiced)
1 handful fresh parsley (chopped)
4 tablespoons organic olive oil (cold pressed)
4 cloves organic garlic (peeled)
1/2 cup fresh avocado (pitted)
1 teaspoon celtic sea salt
1/4 teaspoon ground cumin
1/4 cup raw organic tahini

Place all in food processor until desired consistency. Add water to thin. Keep refrigerated in a sealed container.
Optional-Garnish with organic pine nuts and organic sun-dried tomatoes

Footnotes

1-http://www.ncbi.nlm.nih.gov/pubmed/25648405

2-http://www.vibrancyuk.com/B12.html

3- http://www.ewg.org/research/dirty-dozen-list-endocrine-disruptors

4- http://www.macleans.ca/culture/fresh-from-the-press/

5-http://www.sugarscience.org/sugar-sweetened-beverages/#.VWpOz2C29U4

6- http://www.vegkitchen.com/nutrition/animal-protein-vs-plant-based-protein/?print=pdf

7- http://tinyurl.com/287p2xz

8- http://www.ohp.com/Labels_MSDS/PDF/cycocel_msds.pdf

9- http://www.cspinet.org/new/201102161.html

10- http://www.cbsnews.com/pictures/consumer-reports-spotlights-arsenic-lead-in-10-juices/

11- http://youtu.be/AftZshnP8fs

12- http://www.ncbi.nlm.nih.gov/pubmed/17882683

13-http://www.fda.gov/ForConsumers/ConsumerUpdates/ucm363069.htm

14- http://www.livestrong.com/article/409150-gluten-found-in-gluten-free-products/

15- http://care.diabetesjournals.org/content/26/8/2442.full

16- https://bitesizepieceseducator.files.wordpress.com/2015/04/additives-to-subtract-salad-dressing.pdf

17- http://paleofuture.gizmodo.com/synthetic-hamburgers-are-the-future-and-have-been-for-1029060659food

18- http://www.ncbi.nlm.nih.gov/pmc/articles/PMC1974804/

19- http://listverse.com/2015/03/15/10-bizarre-food-scams-that-could-only-happen-in-china/ see also https://youtu.be/mT-dLoxl7o8

20- http://ajcn.nutrition.org/content/95/2/283.full

21- http://www.cspinet.org/new/201511091.html

22- http://www.ncbi.nlm.nih.gov/pubmed/20424937

23-http://www.eurekalert.org/pub_releases/2016-02/waeh-sdi021216.php

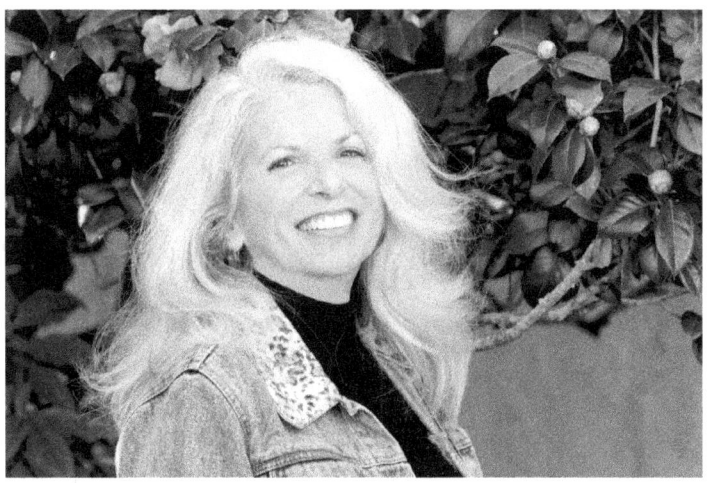

About the Author

Connie Rogers is a Certified Integrative Nutritional Holistic Health Coach, Brain/Gut Coach, Certified Cosmetologist and Skin Health Expert for over 38 years, Gluten-Free Practitioner, Reiki Master, Wellness Blogger, Researcher, Published Author of Path to a Healthy Mind & Body.[5] Accredited through American Association of Drugless Practitioners and Owner of bitesizepieces.net and www.weightlossforlifechange.com Changing the world one story at a time by getting the toxins out, one toxin at a time. Connie's philosophy is that health and wellness are established with proper nutrition, fitness, and awareness. She takes a natural and holistic, common sense approach to rebuilding well-being from the ground up.

---

[5] www.amazon.com/gp/product/0692566066?

Connie's Approach

Nutrition: eat foods that make your whole body smile, not just your taste buds! The right food choices are key to your long-term health, sustainable weight loss, and a powerful immune system. Nutrition and energy go hand and hand. Energy isn't something you lose, it's something you gain when you take the time for self-care.

Exercise: get moving for optimal health and longevity! Find your personal moves that are right for you and be motivated to create lasting strength, agility and stamina.

Spiritual: your thoughts and feelings can be a powerful ally to your healthy body – or its worst enemy. Balance your emotional world for happiness that begins from the inside out.

Mental / Personal Development: discover the facts and dispel the myths that mislead us about our options in life. Get empowered with new skills and the knowledge offered to you from my services, with the correct information.

Environmental: include the world around you into a balanced life with green living choices. Learn how you can make a difference in the wellbeing of your family and friends.

Find your balance and join Connie's program, "21 Steps toward Metabolic Health" https://bitesizepieces.leadpages.co/15-ways-to-metabolic-health/

Connect here: faces@vail.net

You can purchase Connie's Book- Path to a Healthy Mind & Body on Amazon here: http://www.amazon.com/gp/product/0692566066?

DISCLAIMER

The content of this book is for general instruction only.

Each person's physical, emotional, and spiritual condition

is unique. The instruction in this book is not intended to

replace or interrupt the reader's relationship with a

physician or other professional. Please consult your doctor

for matters pertaining to your specific health and dietary needs.